NORMALIZE NURTURING U

A SELF-CARE GUIDE FOR BLACK WOMEN

PAULA MARIE

BlackGirlsDoPilates2

Copyright ©2024

All rights reserved. No part of this book may be used or reproduced without the written permission of the author.

First Edition.

BlackGirlsDoPilates2

ISBN: 979-8-218-42716-0

Printed in USA

TABLE OF CONTENTS

CHAPTER 1 UNDERSTANDING SELF CARE 1

CHAPTER 2 THE IMPACT OF STRESS ON BLACK WOMEN'S HEALTH 9

CHAPTER 3 IDENTIFYING YOUR NEEDS 15

CHAPTER 4 NURTURING YOUR BODY 21

CHAPTER 5 NURTURING YOUR MIND 27

CHAPTER 6 NURTURING YOUR SPIRIT 33

CHAPTER 7 NURTURING YOUR RELATIONSHIPS 39

CHAPTER 8 NURTURING YOUR TIME 45

CHAPTER 9 NURTURING YOUR FUTURE 51

CHAPTER 10 EMBRACING YOUR STRENGTHS .. 57

CHAPTER 11 CULTIVATING JOY AND FULFILLMENT 63

CHAPTER 12   SUSTAINING YOUR SELF CARE JOURNEY 73

CHAPTER 13   EXPLORING SELF CARE RITUALS.79

CHAPTER 14   CONCLUSION 101

Welcome to Normalize Nurturing U, A Self-Care Guide for Black Women. I'm Paula Marie, and I'm thrilled to embark on this journey with you. This book is a celebration of our unique journey as Black women, highlighting the importance of self-care in our lives.

The purpose of this book is to provide you with practical tools and insights to prioritize your well-being. As Black women, we often put the needs of others before our own, leading to burnout and neglect of our health.

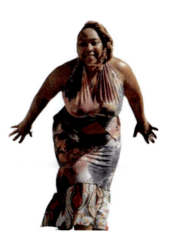

This book aims to empower you to reclaim your time and prioritize self-care as an essential part of your life. Self-care is not selfish; it's necessary for our mental, physical, and emotional health. As Black women, we face unique challenges and stressors that can take a toll on our well-being. By prioritizing self-care, we can nurture ourselves and better support those around us. In this book, you can expect to find practical tips, personal stories, and reflections to inspire and guide you on your self-care journey. You'll discover how to nurture your body, mind, and spirit, and learn to set boundaries and prioritize your needs. I invite you to embrace this book as a companion on your self-care journey. Let's normalize nurturing ourselves and create a culture of self-love and well-being among Black women.

CHAPTER 1

UNDERSTANDING SELF-CARE

A GUIDE FOR BLACK WOMEN

Self-care is a term that's become increasingly popular in recent years, but what does it mean, especially for Black women? In this chapter, we'll explore the concept of self-care, debunk common myths and misconceptions, and discuss why Black women need specific self-care practices tailored to their unique experiences and challenges.

PAULA MARIE

Definition of Self-Care

Self-care is often misunderstood as simply pampering oneself or indulging in luxuries. However, true self-care goes much deeper. At its core, self-care is about taking intentional actions to prioritize your physical, mental, and emotional well-being. It's about recognizing your needs and boundaries, and actively working to meet them.

Self-care can take many forms, from setting aside time for relaxation and leisure activities to seeking professional help when needed. It's about nurturing yourself in a way that promotes overall health and wellness.

For Black women, self-care is especially important due to the unique challenges we face. From systemic racism and microaggressions to the pressure to be strong and resilient, Black women often carry a heavy burden. Self-care offers a way to counteract these challenges and prioritize our own well-being.

Myths and Misconceptions

There are several myths and misconceptions about self-care that can prevent Black women from prioritizing their well-being:

1. Self-care is selfish: This myth suggests that taking care of oneself is selfish or indulgent. In reality, self-care is essential for maintaining your health and well-being, and it can actually make you more effective in caring for others.

2. Self-care is only for the wealthy: Another common misconception is that self-care is only accessible to those who can afford expensive spa treatments or vacations. In reality, self-care can be simple and affordable, such as taking a walk-in nature or practicing deep breathing exercises.

3. Self-care is a luxury: Some people believe that self-care is a luxury that only a few can afford. However, self-care is a necessity for everyone, regardless of their socioeconomic status. It's about prioritizing your well-being and making choices that support your health.

Why Black Women Need Their Own Self-Care Game Plan

Black women face unique challenges and stressors that can impact their health and well-being. From systemic racism and discrimination to the pressure to be strong and resilient, Black women often carry a heavy burden that can take a toll on their physical, mental, and emotional health.

As a result, Black women need specific self-care practices that address these unique challenges. This can include:

1. Healing from racial trauma: Black women may experience racial trauma, which is the psychological and emotional harm caused by experiences of racism and discrimination. Self-care practices that acknowledge and address this trauma can be particularly beneficial.

2. Addressing microaggressions: Black women often face microaggressions, which are subtle, everyday forms of discrimination. Self-care practices that help Black women cope with and respond to these microaggressions can be empowering.

3. Cultivating resilience: Black women have a long history of resilience and strength, but it's important to nurture this resilience through self-care practices. This can include building a strong support network, practicing mindfulness, and setting boundaries.

PAULA MARIE

Practical Self-Care Strategies for Black Women

There are many simple and practical self-care strategies that Black women can incorporate into their daily lives. These include:

- Setting boundaries: Learn to say no to things that drain your energy and prioritize activities that bring you joy and fulfillment.

- Practicing self-compassion: Treat yourself with the same kindness and understanding that you would offer to a friend facing a difficult situation.

- Seeking support: Surround yourself with people who uplift and support you, and don't be afraid to ask for help when you need it.

Incorporating these strategies into your life can help you prioritize your own well-being and lead a more balanced and fulfilling life.

In Summary

Understanding self-care is essential for Black women to prioritize their health and well-being. By debunking myths and misconceptions, and recognizing the need for specific self-care practices, Black women can take proactive steps to nurture themselves and thrive. Remember, self-care is not selfish—it's a necessary act of self-preservation and empowerment.

CHAPTER 2

THE IMPACT OF STRESS ON BLACK WOMEN'S HEALTH

Stress is a natural response to the demands of life, but when it becomes chronic or overwhelming, it can have serious consequences for our health. As Black women, we often face unique stressors that can take a toll on our physical, mental, and emotional well-being. In this chapter, we'll explore the impact of stress on Black women's health and strategies for managing stress effectively.

PAULA MARIE

Understanding Stress

Stress is the body's response to a perceived threat or challenge. When we encounter a stressful situation, our bodies release hormones like cortisol and adrenaline, which trigger the "fight or flight" response. While this response is helpful in the short term, chronic stress can have negative effects on our health.

For Black women, stress can come from many sources, including systemic racism, discrimination, microaggressions, and the pressure to be strong and resilient. These stressors can contribute to a range of health issues, including high blood pressure, heart disease, depression, and anxiety.

One way to do this is by journaling. Writing down your thoughts and feelings can help you see patterns and get a better sense of what's going on inside. You could also chat with a friend, family member, or therapist about what's been on your mind. Sometimes, a fresh perspective can make all the difference.

The Impact of Stress on Health

Chronic stress can have a profound impact on Black women's health. One of the most significant effects of stress is its impact on cardiovascular health. Studies have shown that Black women who experience high levels of stress are at greater risk for heart disease, high blood pressure, and other cardiovascular issues.

Stress can also affect mental health, increasing the risk of depression, anxiety, and other mood disorders. Black women are already at higher risk for these conditions, and chronic stress can further exacerbate these risks.

Additionally, stress can affect our immune systems, making us more susceptible to illness and infection. It can also contribute to inflammation in the body, which is linked to a variety of chronic health conditions.

Keep an eye out for signs like feeling exhausted all the time, snapping at people more than usual, or struggling to concentrate. These could be red flags that you're heading toward burnout. If you notice these signs, don't ignore them. Take some time to rest and recharge, and don't be afraid to ask for help if you need it.

Strategies for Managing Stress

Managing stress effectively is essential for maintaining our health and well-being. While we may not be able to eliminate stress entirely, there are strategies we can use to reduce its impact on our lives:

Self-care: Prioritize self-care activities that help you relax and unwind, such as meditation, yoga, or spending time in nature.

1. Social support: Build a strong support network of friends, family members, and community

members who can offer support and encouragement during stressful times.

2. Healthy lifestyle choices: Eat a balanced diet, exercise regularly, and get plenty of sleep to help your body cope with stress more effectively.

3. Mindfulness: Practice mindfulness techniques such as deep breathing or progressive muscle relaxation to help calm your mind and reduce stress.

4. Professional help: If you're struggling to manage stress on your own, don't hesitate to seek help from a mental health professional who can offer support and guidance.

Summary

Stress is a natural part of life, but when it becomes chronic or overwhelming, it can have serious consequences for our health. As Black women, it's important to recognize the impact of stress on our health and prioritize strategies for managing stress effectively. By taking steps to reduce stress and care for our mental, emotional, and physical well-being, we can improve our overall health and quality of life. Remember, your health is your greatest asset— take care of it.

CHAPTER 3

IDENTIFYING YOUR NEEDS: A ROADMAP TO SELF-CARE

Identifying your needs is the first step towards practicing effective self-care. It involves taking an honest look at your current state, recognizing signs of burnout, and setting realistic self-care goals. In this chapter, we'll explore these key components of self-care and provide strategies for identifying and prioritizing your needs.

Assessing Your Current State

To effectively identify your needs, it's important to assess your current state. This involves taking stock of various aspects of your life, including your physical, mental, and emotional well-being, as well as your relationships, work, and other responsibilities.

One way to assess your current state is to ask yourself the following questions:

- How do I feel physically? Do I have any health concerns or symptoms that need attention?

- How do I feel mentally and emotionally? Am I experiencing stress, anxiety, or other negative emotions?

- How are my relationships? Do I feel supported and connected to others, or do I feel isolated?

- How is my work and other responsibilities impacting my well-being? Am I feeling overwhelmed or burned out?

Recognizing Signs of Burnout

Burnout is a state of physical, emotional, and mental exhaustion caused by prolonged stress or overwhelming responsibilities.

It can manifest in various ways, including:

- Physical symptoms such as fatigue, headaches, or digestive issues
- Emotional symptoms such as irritability, mood swings, or feelings of hopelessness
- Cognitive symptoms such as difficulty concentrating or making decisions
- Behavioral symptoms such as withdrawal from social activities or increased use of substances

Recognizing these signs of burnout is crucial for preventing further health issues and prioritizing self-care.

Setting Self-Care Goals

Once you've assessed your current state and recognized signs of burnout, the next step is to set self-care goals. These goals should be specific, measurable, achievable, relevant, and time-bound (SMART).

Here are some examples of self-care goals:

- Physical self-care: I will exercise for at least 30 minutes three times a week to improve my physical health and energy levels.
- Emotional self-care: I will practice mindfulness meditation for 10 minutes each day to reduce stress and improve my emotional well-being.

- Social self-care: I will schedule regular social activities with friends or family members to improve my social connections and support network.

- Professional self-care: I will set boundaries at work and prioritize tasks to avoid feeling overwhelmed and burned out.

Summary

Identifying your needs is the first step toward practicing effective self-care. By assessing your current state, recognizing signs of burnout, and setting realistic self-care goals, you can prioritize your well-being and take proactive steps to improve your physical, mental, and emotional health. Remember, self-care is not selfish—it's a necessary act of self-preservation and empowerment.

CHAPTER 4

NURTURING YOUR BODY

A COMPREHENSIVE GUIDE TO HEALTH AND WELLNESS

Nurturing your body is essential for overall health and well-being. In this chapter, we'll explore the importance of healthy eating habits, exercise and movement, and skincare tips specifically tailored for Black women. By prioritizing these aspects of self-care, you can enhance your physical health, boost your energy levels, and improve your overall quality of life.

In this chapter, we'll explore ways to nourish our bodies through healthy eating habits, regular exercise, and skincare routines tailored to our unique needs.

Healthy Eating Habits

Healthy eating habits are key to nurturing your body and providing it with the nutrients it needs to function properly. As Black women, it's important to focus on a balanced diet that includes a variety of fruits, vegetables, whole grains, lean proteins, and healthy fats. Here are some tips for maintaining healthy eating habits:

1. Plan your meals: Take the time to plan your meals for the week, and aim to include a variety of nutritious foods in your diet.

2. Cook at home: Cooking at home allows you to control the ingredients in your meals and can help you make healthier choices.

3. Stay hydrated: Drink plenty of water throughout the day to stay hydrated and support your body's functions.

4. Limit processed foods: Try to limit your intake of processed foods, which are often high in unhealthy fats, sugars, and additives.

5. Practice mindful eating: Pay attention to your body's hunger and fullness cues, and eat slowly to fully enjoy and digest your food.

Exercise and Movement

Regular exercise and movement are essential for maintaining a healthy body and mind. Exercise can help improve your cardiovascular health, strengthen your muscles, and boost your mood. As a Black woman, it's important to find activities that you enjoy and that fit into your lifestyle. Here are some tips for incorporating exercise and movement into your routine:

1. Find activities you enjoy: Whether it's dancing, yoga, walking, or playing a sport, find activities that you enjoy and that make you feel good.

2. Make it a habit: Aim to incorporate exercise into your daily routine, whether it's a morning walk, a lunchtime workout, or an evening yoga session.

3. Stay consistent: Consistency is key when it comes to exercise. Try to exercise at least three to four times a week to see the benefits.

4. Listen to your body: Pay attention to how your body feels during and after exercise, and adjust your routine as needed to avoid injury.

Skincare Tips for Black Women

Skincare is an important aspect of nurturing your body, especially for Black women who may have specific skincare needs. Here are some skincare tips for Black women:

1. Moisturize regularly: Black skin tends to be drier than other skin types, so it's important to

moisturize daily to keep your skin hydrated and healthy.

2. Use sunscreen: Despite the misconception that Black skin is not prone to sun damage, it's important to use sunscreen daily to protect your skin from harmful UV rays.

3. Avoid harsh products: Be cautious of using harsh skincare products that can strip your skin of its natural oils. Look for gentle, hydrating products instead.

4. Stay hydrated: Drinking plenty of water can help keep your skin hydrated from the inside out.

PAULA MARIE

Summary

Nurturing your body is an essential part of self-care. By prioritizing healthy eating, regular exercise, and a skincare routine tailored to your needs, you can support your physical health and well-being. As Black women, it's important to remember that self-care is not selfish—it's an investment in your health and happiness. So, take the time to nourish your body and show it the love it deserves.

CHAPTER 5

NURTURING YOUR MIND
STRATEGIES FOR YOUR WELL-BEING

Nurturing your mind is essential for overall health and well-being. In this chapter, we'll explore stress management techniques, mental health awareness, and strategies for cultivating a positive mindset. By prioritizing your mental health, you can improve your mood, reduce stress, and enhance your overall quality of life.

PAULA MARIE

Stress Management Techniques

Stress is a natural part of life, but too much stress can take a toll on your mental and physical health. It's important to have effective stress management techniques to help you cope with stress. Here are some strategies you can use:

1. Practice relaxation techniques: Techniques such as deep breathing, meditation, and yoga can help calm your mind and reduce stress levels.

2. Exercise regularly: Physical activity can help reduce stress and improve your mood. Aim for at least 30 minutes of moderate exercise most days of the week.

3. Get enough sleep: Lack of sleep can contribute to stress and affect your mood.

4. Aim for 7-9 hours of quality sleep each night.

5. Connect with others: Talking to friends, family, or a therapist can help you feel supported and reduce feelings of stress and anxiety.

6. Manage your time effectively: Prioritize your tasks and avoid overcommitting yourself to reduce feelings of being overwhelmed.

Mental Health Awareness

Mental health awareness is essential for recognizing when you or someone you know may be struggling with mental health issues. Common mental health disorders such as depression, anxiety, and PTSD are prevalent among Black women, and it's important to seek help if you're experiencing symptoms. Here are some signs that you may need to seek help:

1. Persistent feelings of sadness or hopelessness

2. Loss of interest in activities you once enjoyed

3. Changes in appetite or sleep patterns

4. Difficulty concentrating or making decisions
5. Increased use of alcohol or drugs
6. Thoughts of self-harm or suicide If you or someone you know is experiencing these symptoms, it's important to seek help from a mental health professional.

Cultivating a Positive Mindset

Cultivating a positive mindset can help improve your mental health and overall well-being. Here are some strategies for cultivating a positive mindset:

1. Practice gratitude: Take time each day to reflect on the things you're grateful for. This can help shift your focus from negative to positive thoughts.
2. Challenge negative thoughts: When you notice negative thoughts, challenge them with more realistic and positive thoughts.

3. Surround yourself with positivity: Spend time with people who uplift and support you, and engage in activities that bring you joy and fulfillment.

4. Practice self-compassion: Treat yourself with kindness and understanding, especially during difficult times.

Summary

Nurturing your mind is an essential part of self-care. By managing stress, promoting mental health awareness, and cultivating a positive mindset, you can support your mental health and well-being. As Black women, it's important to prioritize your mental health and seek help if you need it. Remember, taking care of your mind is not selfish—it's an investment in your health and happiness.

CHAPTER 6

NURTURING YOUR SPIRIT

CULTIVATING INNER PEACE AND SPIRITUAL CONNECTION

Nurturing your spirit is essential for overall well-being and inner peace. In this chapter, we'll explore practices for finding inner peace, practicing gratitude, and connecting with your spiritual side. By nurturing your spirit, you can cultivate a sense of purpose, meaning, and fulfillment in your life.

PAULA MARIE

Finding Inner Peace

Inner peace is a state of calmness and tranquility that comes from within. It's about finding balance and harmony in your life, even amid challenges and chaos. Here are some practices for finding inner peace:

1. Meditation: Meditation is a powerful tool for calming the mind and finding inner peace. Set aside time each day to sit quietly and focus on your breath or a mantra.

2. Mindfulness: Mindfulness is the practice of being present in the moment and fully engaged in what you're doing. Practice mindfulness in your daily activities, such as eating or walking.

3. Nature walks: Spending time in nature can help you connect with the world around you and find a sense of peace and calm.

4. Yoga: Yoga combines physical postures, breathing techniques, and meditation to help you find balance and inner peace.

Practicing Gratitude

Practicing gratitude is a powerful way to nurture your spirit and shift your focus from what you lack to what you have. Here are some ways to practice gratitude:

1. Keep a gratitude journal: Each day, write down three things you're grateful for. This simple practice can help you cultivate a more positive outlook on life.

2. Express gratitude to others: Take the time to thank the people in your life who have helped or supported you. This can strengthen your relationships and increase your sense of connection.

3. Count your blessings: When you're feeling down or discouraged, take a moment to count

your blessings and remind yourself of all the good things in your life.

Connecting with Your Spiritual Side

Spirituality is a deeply personal and individual experience, but it can provide a sense of meaning, purpose, and connection to something greater than yourself. Here are some ways to connect with your spiritual side:

1. Explore different spiritual practices: Whether it's through prayer, meditation, or attending religious services, explore different spiritual practices to find what resonates with you.

2. Connect with others: Joining a spiritual community or group can provide support, guidance, and a sense of belonging.

3. Reflect on your values and beliefs: Take time to reflect on what's truly important to you and how your values and beliefs shape your life.

Summary

Nurturing your spirit is an essential part of selfcare. By finding inner peace, practicing gratitude, and connecting with your spiritual side, you can cultivate a sense of peace and fulfillment in your life. As Black women, it's important to prioritize your spiritual well-being and make time for practices that nourish your spirit. Remember, taking care of your spirit is not selfish—it's a vital part of living a balanced and fulfilling life.

CHAPTER 7

NURTURING YOUR RELATIONSHIPS

BUILDING SUPPORTIVE BONDS AND SETTING HEALTHY BOUNDARIES

Nurturing your relationships is essential for overall well-being and happiness. In this chapter, we'll explore strategies for building supportive relationships, setting healthy boundaries, and balancing the various relationships in your life. By prioritizing your relationships and investing in meaningful connections, you can enhance your social support network and improve your overall quality of life.

Building Supportive Relationships

Supportive relationships are key to emotional well-being and resilience. These relationships provide a sense of belonging, validation, and support during challenging times. Here are some strategies for building supportive relationships:

1. Be present: Show up for your loved ones and be present in their lives. Listen actively, offer support, and be there when they need you.

2. Communicate openly: Effective communication is crucial for building supportive relationships. Be honest, express your needs and feelings, and listen to the needs and feelings of others.

3. Show appreciation: Take the time to express gratitude and appreciation for the people in your life. Small gestures of kindness can strengthen your relationships and deepen your connections.

4. Be a good friend: Be a supportive and reliable friend to others. Offer your help, lend a listening ear, and celebrate their successes.

Setting Boundaries

Setting healthy boundaries is essential for maintaining healthy relationships and protecting your well-being. Boundaries help define what is acceptable and unacceptable behavior in your relationships. Here are some tips for setting boundaries:

1. *Identify your limits:* Take the time to identify your physical, emotional, and mental limits in your relationships.

2. *Communicate your boundaries:* Clearly communicate your boundaries to others in a calm and assertive manner. Be firm and consistent in enforcing your boundaries.

3. *Respect others' boundaries:* Respect the boundaries of others and avoid pressuring them to go beyond their comfort zone.

Balancing Family, Friendships, and Romantic Relationships

Balancing the various relationships in your life can be challenging, but it's important to prioritize each relationship based on its significance and impact on your well-being. Here are some tips for balancing family, friendships, and romantic relationships:

1. *Prioritize self-care:* Take care of yourself physically, emotionally, and mentally so that you can be fully present in your relationships.

2. *Manage your time effectively:* Prioritize your relationships based on their importance and allocate time accordingly.

3. *Communicate openly:* Communicate with your loved ones about your commitments and priorities to avoid misunderstandings and conflicts.

Summary

Nurturing your relationships is essential for your overall well-being and happiness. By building supportive relationships, setting healthy boundaries, and balancing the various relationships in your life, you can enhance your social support network and improve your overall quality of life. Remember, your relationships are a source of strength and joy—nurture them and watch them flourish

CHAPTER 8

NURTURING YOUR TIME

STRATEGIES FOR TIME MANAGEMENT AND SELF-CARE

Nurturing your time is crucial for maintaining balance and well-being in your life. In this chapter, we'll explore effective time management strategies, the importance of prioritizing self-care in your schedule, and how to say no to overcommitment. By managing your time effectively and prioritizing self-care, you can reduce stress, increase productivity, and improve your overall quality of life.

PAULA MARIE

Time Management Strategies

Effective time management is key to making the most of your time and achieving your goals. Here are some strategies for managing your time effectively:

1. *Set goals:* Clearly define your goals and priorities to help you stay focused and motivated.

2. *Prioritize tasks:* Identify the most important tasks and tackle them first to ensure they get done.

3. *Use a planner or calendar:* Use a planner or calendar to schedule your tasks and appointments, and keep track of deadlines.

4. *Break tasks into smaller steps:* Break large tasks into smaller, more manageable steps to avoid feeling overwhelmed.

5. *Limit distractions:* Identify and eliminate distractions that may prevent you from staying focused on your tasks.

Prioritizing Self-Care in Your Schedule

Self-care is essential for maintaining your physical, mental, and emotional well-being. It's important to prioritize self-care in your schedule to ensure you're taking care of yourself. Here are some ways to prioritize self-care in your schedule:

1. *Schedule self-care activities:* Set aside time in your schedule for activities that nourish your mind, body, and soul, such as exercise, meditation, or hobbies.

2. *Set boundaries:* Learn to say no to commitments that interfere with your selfcare routine and prioritize activities that recharge you.

3. *Practice mindfulness:* Stay present in the moment and focus on what you're doing to reduce stress and improve your overall wellbeing.

PAULA MARIE

Saying No to Overcommitment

Learning to say no is an important skill that can help you avoid overcommitment and maintain balance in your life. Here are some tips for saying no effectively:

1. *Be honest and respectful:* Politely decline requests and explain your reasons for saying no.

2. *Offer alternatives:* If possible, offer alternatives or compromises that may meet the other person's needs without overcommitting yourself.

3. *Practice self-compassion:* Remember that it's okay to say no and prioritize your own needs and well-being.

Conclusion

Nurturing your time is an essential part of self-care. By managing your time effectively, prioritizing self-care, and learning to say no to overcommitment, you can create a more balanced and fulfilling life. As Black women, it's important to value your time and use it wisely. Remember, you deserve to prioritize your own needs and make time for the things that matter most to you.

CHAPTER 9

NURTURING YOUR FUTURE

SETTING LONG-TERM SELF-CARE GOALS AND CELEBRATING YOUR PROGRESS

Nurturing your future involves setting long-term self-care goals, overcoming obstacles, and celebrating your progress along the way. In this chapter, we'll explore strategies for setting meaningful goals, overcoming common obstacles, and celebrating your achievements. By nurturing your future, you can create a life filled with health, happiness, and fulfillment.

Setting Long-Term Self-Care Goals

Setting long-term self-care goals is essential for creating a roadmap to a healthier, happier life. When setting these goals, it's important to make them specific, measurable, achievable, relevant, and time-bound (SMART).

Here are some tips for setting long-term selfcare goals:

1. *Reflect on your values and priorities:* Consider what's truly important to you and how you want to prioritize your well-being in the long term.

2. *Break goals into smaller steps:* Break down your long-term goals into smaller, more manageable steps to make them less daunting.

3. *Stay flexible:* Be open to adjusting your goals as needed based on your progress and changing circumstances.

Overcoming Obstacles

Obstacles are a natural part of the journey to achieving your goals. It's important to anticipate and prepare for obstacles so you can overcome them when they arise.

Here are some common obstacles to self-care and strategies for overcoming them:

1. *Lack of time:* Prioritize self-care in your schedule and make it a non-negotiable part of your routine.

2. *Lack of motivation:* Remind yourself of your long-term goals and the benefits of self-care, and seek support from friends, family, or a therapist if needed.

3. *Burnout:* Recognize the signs of burnout and take proactive steps to prevent it, such as setting boundaries and practicing self-care regularly.

Celebrating Your Progress

Celebrating your progress is an important part of nurturing your future and staying motivated. Celebrating small wins along the way can help you stay motivated and focused on your longterm goals.

Here are some ways to celebrate your progress:

1. *Acknowledge your achievements:* Take the time to acknowledge and celebrate your achievements, no matter how small.

2. *Reward yourself:* Treat yourself to something special as a reward for reaching a milestone or achieving a goal.

3. *Share your success:* Share your success with others and celebrate with friends, family, or colleagues who have supported you along the way.

Conclusion

Nurturing your future involves setting long-term self-care goals, overcoming obstacles, and celebrating your progress. By setting meaningful goals, overcoming obstacles, and celebrating your achievements, you can create a life filled with health, happiness, and fulfillment.

Remember, your future is in your hands—nurture it, embrace it, and celebrate it

CHAPTER 10

EMBRACING YOUR STRENGTHS

As Black women, we are often praised for our strength and resilience in the face of adversity. While these qualities are undoubtedly valuable, it's also important to recognize and embrace our other strengths—our creativity, intelligence, compassion, and more. In this chapter, we'll explore the concept of strengths-based self-care and how embracing our strengths can enhance our well-being.

PAULA MARIE

Understanding Strengths-Based Self Care

Strengths-based self-care is an approach to self-care that focuses on identifying and leveraging your unique strengths to promote your well-being. Instead of focusing solely on fixing your weaknesses or overcoming challenges, strength-based self-care encourages you to recognize and celebrate the things that make you strong and resilient.

Identifying Your Strengths

One way to embrace your strengths is by identifying them. Take some time to reflect on the qualities that you admire in yourself and that others have complimented you on. These could be things like your creativity, your ability to empathize with others, your sense of humor, or your resilience in the face of adversity. You can also use tools like the VIA Survey of Character Strengths to help you identify your strengths. This survey identifies 24 universal character strengths, such as bravery, kindness, and honesty, and can provide insight into your own unique strengths.

Celebrating Your Strengths

Once you've identified your strengths, it's important to celebrate them. Take pride in the things that make you strong and unique. This could involve acknowledging your strengths in a journal, sharing them with a friend, or simply taking a moment to appreciate them yourself.

PAULA MARIE

Using Your Strengths in Self-Care

One of the key benefits of embracing your strengths is that it can enhance your self-care practices. For example, if one of your strengths is creativity, you might incorporate creative activities like painting, writing, or crafting into your self-care routine. If your strength is empathy, you might focus on connecting with others and building supportive relationships as part of your self-care.

Overcoming Challenges

While embracing your strengths can be empowering, it's also important to recognize that you may face challenges along the way. Internalized racism, societal expectations, and self-doubt can all undermine your efforts to embrace your strengths. It's important to be gentle with yourself and to practice selfcompassion as you navigate these challenges.

Conclusion

Embracing your strengths is a powerful form of self-care that can enhance your well-being and resilience. By recognizing and celebrating the things that make you strong and unique, you can cultivate a sense of empowerment and selfworth. As Black women, it's important to embrace our strengths as a source of pride and resilience in the face of adversity. Remember, you are strong, you are capable, and you are deserving of all the love and care in the world.

CHAPTER 11

CULTIVATING JOY AND FULFILLMENT

In the midst of life's challenges and responsibilities, it's important to make time for joy and fulfillment. As Black women, we often prioritize the needs of others over our own, but it's essential to prioritize our own happiness and well-being. In this chapter, we'll explore ways to cultivate joy and fulfillment in your life, even in the face of adversity.

PAULA MARIE

Finding Joy in Everyday Moments

Joy can be found in the simplest of moments, from a beautiful sunset to a heartfelt conversation with a loved one. As Black women, it's important to slow down and savor these moments, rather than constantly striving for more. Take time each day to notice and appreciate the beauty and joy that surrounds you.

One way to find joy in everyday moments is to practice mindfulness. Mindfulness involves being fully present in the moment, without judgment. Take a few minutes each day to pause and notice your surroundings. Pay attention to the sights, sounds, and sensations around you. This can help you cultivate a greater sense of appreciation for the world around you and find joy in the present moment.

NORMALIZE NURTURING U

Practicing Gratitude

Practicing gratitude is another powerful way to cultivate joy and fulfillment. Take time each day to reflect on the things you're grateful for, whether it's a supportive friend, a delicious meal, or a moment of peace and quiet. Gratitude can help shift your focus from what you lack to what you have, increasing your overall sense of wellbeing.

One way to practice gratitude is to keep a gratitude journal. Each day, write down three things you're grateful for. They can be big or small, from a kind gesture from a stranger to a major accomplishment at work. By focusing on the positive aspects of your life, you can cultivate a sense of abundance and contentment.

PAULA MARIE

Engaging in Activities That Bring You Joy

Engaging in activities that bring you joy is another important aspect of cultivating fulfillment. Whether it's dancing, painting, gardening, or cooking, make time for activities that nourish your soul and bring you happiness. These activities can help you recharge and rejuvenate, making it easier to face life's challenges with a positive mindset.

Think about the activities that bring you joy and make a commitment to incorporate them into your life regularly. Schedule time for these activities just as you would for any other important commitment. Whether it's a weekly dance class or a daily walk in nature, prioritize activities that bring you joy and make you feel alive.

Building Meaningful Connections

Building meaningful connections with others is essential for cultivating joy and fulfillment. As Black women, we often find strength and support in our relationships with family, friends, and community. Take time to nurture these relationships and build new connections with like-minded individuals who uplift and inspire you.

One way to build meaningful connections is to participate in community activities or groups that align with your interests and values. Whether it's volunteering for a cause you're passionate about or joining a book club, seek out opportunities to connect with others who share your passions and values. These connections can provide a sense of belonging and support that can enhance your overall well-being.

PAULA MARIE

Setting Goals That Align With Your Values

Setting goals that align with your values is another important aspect of cultivating fulfillment. Take some time to reflect on what matters most to you and set goals that reflect those values. Whether it's advancing in your career, starting a family, or giving back to your community, setting meaningful goals can give you a sense of purpose and fulfillment.

When setting goals, it's important to make sure they are specific, measurable, attainable, relevant, and time-bound (SMART). This can help you stay focused and motivated as you work towards achieving your goals. Break your goals down into smaller, manageable steps and celebrate your progress along the way.

NORMALIZE NURTURING U

Embracing Your Authentic Self

Finally, embracing your authentic self is essential for cultivating joy and fulfillment. As Black women, we often face societal pressures to conform to certain standards of beauty, success, and behavior. It's important to resist these pressures and embrace who you truly are, flaws and all. Celebrate your uniqueness and honor your own path in life.

One way to embrace your authentic self is to practice self-acceptance. This means accepting yourself as you are, without judgment or criticism. Recognize that you are worthy of love and respect just as you are, and treat yourself with the same kindness and compassion that you would offer to a friend.

PAULA MARIE

Overcoming Challenges

While cultivating joy and fulfillment can be a rewarding journey, it's important to recognize that you may face challenges along the way. Internalized racism, societal expectations, and self-doubt can all undermine your efforts to cultivate joy and fulfillment. It's important to be gentle with yourself and to practice selfcompassion as you navigate these challenges.

One way to overcome these challenges is to seek support from others. Whether it's friends, family, or a therapist, having a support system in place can help you navigate difficult times and stay on track with your goals. Remember, it's okay to ask for help when you need it, and you don't have to face challenges alone.

Summary

Cultivating joy and fulfillment is an ongoing process that requires intention and effort. By finding joy in everyday moments, practicing gratitude, engaging in activities that bring you joy, building meaningful connections, setting goals that align with your values, and embracing your authentic self, you can create a life that is rich and fulfilling.

As Black women, it's important to prioritize your own happiness and well-being, and to make time for the things that bring you joy. Remember, you deserve to live a life that is joyful, fulfilling, and true to who you are.

CHAPTER 12

SUSTAINING YOUR SELF-CARE JOURNEY

Embarking on a journey of self-care is a powerful step towards living a more fulfilling and balanced life. However, sustaining this journey over time can be challenging, especially in the face of life's ups and downs. In this chapter, we'll explore strategies for maintaining your self-care practices and overcoming obstacles that may arise along the way.

PAULA MARIE

Reflecting on Your Progress

As you continue on your self-care journey, take time to reflect on your progress and celebrate your successes. Reflecting on how far you've come can help you stay motivated and inspired to continue your self-care practices. Consider keeping a journal to track your progress and write down any insights or discoveries you've made along the way.

Adapting to Life Changes

Life is constantly changing, and it's important to adapt your self-care practices to meet your evolving needs. As Black women, we often face unique challenges and responsibilities that can impact our self-care routines. Whether it's a change in your work schedule, a new family dynamic, or a shift in your health, be flexible and willing to adjust your self-care practices as needed.

One way to adapt to life changes is to be proactive about planning ahead. Anticipate potential challenges or disruptions to your selfcare routine and brainstorm ways to address them. For example, if you know you'll have a busy week at work, plan ahead by scheduling shorter self-care activities or finding ways to incorporate self-care into your daily routine.

Creating a Support System

Having a support system in place can be instrumental in sustaining your self-care journey. Surround yourself with people who support and encourage your self-care efforts. Whether it's friends, family members, or a support group, having people to turn to during difficult times can help you stay on track with your self-care practices.

If you don't have a support system in place, consider joining a community or group that shares your interests or values. Online communities can also be a valuable source of support and encouragement. Remember, you don't have to go through your self-care journey alone—seeking support from others can help you stay motivated and inspired.

Managing Setbacks

Despite your best efforts, you may encounter setbacks on your self-care journey. Whether it's a lapse in your self-care routine or a challenging life event, it's important to approach setbacks with compassion and resilience. Remember that setbacks are a natural part of any journey, and they don't define your progress or success.

One way to manage setbacks is to practice self-compassion. Treat yourself with the same kindness and understanding that you would offer to a friend facing a similar challenge. Instead of dwelling on the setback, focus on what you can learn from the experience and how you can move forward in a positive way.

Revisiting Your Self-Care Plan

Periodically revisiting your self-care plan can help you stay on track and ensure that your selfcare practices continue to meet your needs. As you reflect on your progress and identify areas for improvement, consider updating your selfcare plan to reflect any changes or insights you've gained along the way.

When revisiting your self-care plan, consider the following questions:

- Are my self-care practices still serving me well, or do I need to make adjustments? • Are there any new self-care practices I'd like to incorporate into my routine?

- How can I continue to prioritize self-care in the face of life's challenges and responsibilities?

Conclusion

Sustaining your self-care journey is a lifelong process that requires commitment, flexibility, and self-compassion. By reflecting on your progress, adapting to life changes, creating a support system, managing setbacks, and revisiting your self-care plan regularly, you can maintain your self-care practices and continue to prioritize your well-being. As Black women, it's important to recognize that self-care is not selfish—it's an essential part of living a balanced and fulfilling life. Remember, you deserve to prioritize your own well-being and happiness.

CHAPTER 13

EXPLORING SELF-CARE RITUALS

Self-care has become a buzzword in recent years, often associated with indulgent spa days or luxurious bubble baths. While these practices can certainly be part of self-care, they only scratch the surface of what it truly entails. Self-care is about intentionally taking care of oneself, not just physically but also emotionally, mentally, and spiritually. It is a holistic approach to well-being that acknowledges the interconnectedness of these aspects of our lives.

Self-care rituals, in particular, are the regular practices or routines that individuals engage in to nurture and nourish themselves. These rituals can vary widely from person to person, influenced by cultural background, personal preferences, and life experiences. For Black women, in particular, self-care rituals can be deeply rooted in cultural traditions and familial customs, making them both unique and significant.

I surveyed over 500 Black women and asked them to give their self-care rituals. In this chapter, we will explore the diverse ways in which they choose to prioritize their well-being. Through these insights, we hope to not only highlight the importance of self-care for Black women but also inspire others to embrace their own self-care journeys.

Defining Self-Care Rituals

Before we begin, it is important to define what we mean by self-care rituals. While the term "self-care" is often used broadly, encompassing everything from taking a mental health day to practicing gratitude, self-care rituals specifically refer to the intentional and regular practices that individuals engage in to promote their well-being.

These rituals can encompass a wide range of activities, from the mundane to the extraordinary. They can be as simple as a daily skincare routine or as elaborate as a weekend getaway. What sets self-care rituals apart is the intention behind them – they are not just activities that we do out of habit or obligation, but rather, they are actions that we consciously choose to engage in because we know they contribute to our overall well-being.

Self-care rituals can also be highly personalized, reflecting the unique needs and preferences of each individual. What works for one person may not work for another, and that's perfectly okay. The key is to find what resonates with you and brings you a sense of peace, joy, and rejuvenation.

This chapter offers a glimpse into the myriad ways in which Black women prioritize their self-care. Through this list, we hope to inspire others to discover and embrace their own self-care rituals, recognizing that self-care is not a luxury but a necessity for overall well-being.

NORMALIZE NURTURING U

Here's a list of 50 self-care rituals for Black women by Black women.

1. Morning Affirmations
    - *Description:* Start your day with positive affirmations to set the tone for the day.
    - *Benefits:* Increases self-confidence, reduces stress, improves focus, enhances mood.
2. Pilates Practice
    - *Description:* Engage in a regular Pilates practice to improve flexibility, reduce stress, and promote relaxation and mindfulness.
    - *Benefits:* Improves flexibility, reduces stress, promotes relaxation, enhances muscle tone and strength.

3. Reading for Pleasure

    - *Description:* Set aside time to read books that you enjoy.

    - *Benefits:* Reduces stress, improves focus and concentration, enhances empathy and emotional intelligence.

4. Vacuuming

    - *Description:* Engage in vacuuming your living space.

    - *Benefits:* Improves indoor air quality by removing dust and allergens, enhances cleanliness and hygiene, provides a sense of accomplishment, promotes physical activity and movement.

5. Spa Day at Home

    - *Description*: Create a spa-like atmosphere at home with candles, soothing music, and pampering treatments.

- *Benefits:* Promotes relaxation, reduces muscle tension, improves skin health, enhances mental clarity.

6. Nature Walks

    - *Description:* Spend time in nature to reduce stress, improve mood, and boost overall well-being.
    - *Benefits:* Reduces stress, boosts mood, improves cardiovascular health, enhances immune function.

7. Creative Writing

    - *Description:* Express your thoughts and emotions through creative writing.
    - *Benefits:* Improves emotional well-being, enhances creativity, reduces stress, promotes self-expression.

8. Mindful Breathing

    - *Description:* Practice deep breathing exercises to reduce stress, improve focus, and promote relaxation.
    - *Benefits:* Reduces stress, improves lung function, enhances focus and concentration, promotes relaxation.

9. Meal Prep

    - *Description:* Dedicate time to prepare and portion meals in advance.
    - *Benefits:* Promotes healthy eating habits, saves time during the week, reduces reliance on unhealthy convenience foods, allows for better portion control, supports weight management goals.

10. Dance Therapy

    - *Description:* Dance to your favorite music to release tension, improve mood, and boost energy levels.

- *Benefits:* Improves cardiovascular health, boosts mood, enhances flexibility and coordination, reduces stress.

11. Journaling

    - *Description:* Write in a journal to reflect on your thoughts and emotions.
    - *Benefits:* Improves mental health, enhances self-awareness, reduces stress, promotes emotional healing.

12. Healthy Cooking

    - *Description:* Prepare nutritious meals using fresh ingredients.
    - *Benefits:* Improves nutrition, boosts energy levels, supports weight management, enhances mood.

13. Crystal Meditation

    - *Description:* Meditate with crystals.

    - *Benefits:* Enhances meditation practice, balances energy, promotes relaxation, reduces stress.

14. Energy Cleansing

    - *Description:* Use sage or palo santo to cleanse your space and energy.

    - *Benefits:* Clears negative energy, promotes positivity, enhances spiritual well-being, reduces stress.

15. Positive Visualization

    - *Description:* Visualize positive outcomes for your goals.

    - *Benefits:* Increases motivation, reduces stress, enhances focus, improves self-confidence.

16. Bird Watching

    - *Description:* Spend time observing birds in their natural habitat.

    - *Benefits:* Reduces stress, promotes mindfulness, connects you with nature, enhances mood.

17. Cleaning

    - *Description:* Engage in cleaning your living space.

    - *Benefits:* Improves mood, reduces stress, enhances productivity, promotes a sense of accomplishment.

18. Bubble Bath

    - *Description:* Take a relaxing bath with bubble bath or bath salts.

    - *Benefits:* Promotes relaxation, reduces muscle tension, improves skin health, enhances mental clarity.

19. Coffee Shops

- *Description:* Visit coffee shops for a cozy and relaxing atmosphere.

- *Benefits:* Provides a change of environment, enhances mood, promotes social interactions, boosts productivity.

20. Coloring

- *Description:* Engage in coloring activities.

- *Benefits:* Reduces stress and anxiety, improves focus and concentration, promotes relaxation, enhances creativity.

21. Dancing

- *Description:* Dance to your favorite music.

- *Benefits:* Improves cardiovascular health, boosts mood, enhances flexibility and coordination, reduces stress.

22. Exercise

    - *Description:* Engage in regular physical activity.
    - *Benefits:* Improves overall health, boosts mood, reduces stress, enhances energy levels.

23. Exfoliate

    - *Description:* Use exfoliating products to remove dead skin cells.
    - *Benefits:* Improves skin texture, promotes cell turnover, enhances skin radiance, prevents clogged pores.

24. Face Mask

    - *Description:* Apply a face mask to nourish and hydrate your skin.
    - *Benefits:* Improves skin hydration, reduces acne and blemishes, enhances skin clarity, promotes relaxation.

25. Facial Steaming

- *Description:* Steam your face to open pores and promote skin health.
- *Benefits:* Cleanses pores, improves circulation, enhances skin radiance, promotes relaxation.

26. Flower Baths

- *Description:* Take a bath with fresh flowers.
- *Benefits:* Promotes relaxation, enhances mood, improves skin health, provides aromatherapy benefits.

27. Flower Arrangement

- *Description:* Arrange flowers as a creative and soothing activity.
- *Benefits:* Enhances creativity, reduces stress, promotes mindfulness, boosts mood.

28. Foot Massage

    - *Description:* Give yourself a foot massage or visit a professional.

    - *Benefits:* Relieves foot pain and tension, promotes relaxation, improves circulation, enhances mood.

29. Therapy

    - *Description:* Attend therapy sessions to work through emotional issues.

    - *Benefits:* Improves mental health, enhances self-awareness, reduces stress, promotes emotional healing.

30. Ginger Shots

    - *Description:* Take ginger shots for their health benefits.

    - *Benefits:* Boosts immune system, reduces inflammation, aids in digestion, improves circulation.

31. Hot Tea

- *Description:* Enjoy a cup of hot tea.

- *Benefits:* Promotes relaxation, enhances hydration, provides antioxidants, improves digestion.

32. Sit at the Beach or by a Lake

- *Description:* Spend time sitting and enjoying the view at the beach or by a lake.

- *Benefits:* Reduces stress, promotes relaxation, connects you with nature, enhances mood.

33. Intentional Prayer

- *Description:* Engage in prayer with intention and focus.

- *Benefits:* Improves spiritual well-being, reduces stress, enhances mindfulness, promotes a sense of peace.

34. Intermittent Fasting

    - *Description:* Practice intermittent fasting as a dietary approach.
    - *Benefits:* Promotes weight loss, improves metabolic health, enhances brain function, may reduce inflammation.

35. Listening to Subliminals

    - *Description:* Listen to subliminal audio tracks for various purposes (e.g., relaxation, motivation).
    - *Benefits:* Promotes relaxation, enhances mood, improves focus, supports personal development goals.

36. Long Walks

    - *Description:* Take long walks in nature or around your neighborhood.
    - *Benefits:* Reduces stress, boosts mood, improves cardiovascular health, enhances mental clarity.

37. Crochet

- *Description:* Engage in crocheting as a creative and relaxing activity.
- *Benefits:* Reduces stress, enhances creativity, promotes mindfulness, boosts mood.

38. Skin Care

- *Description:* Follow a regular skin care routine.
- *Benefits:* Improves skin health, promotes relaxation, enhances self-care routine, boosts self-confidence.

39. Nails

- *Description:* Care for your nails by trimming, shaping, and painting them.
- *Benefits:* Improves nail health, enhances appearance, promotes relaxation, boosts self-confidence.

40. Naps

- *Description:* Take short naps during the day.
- *Benefits:* Improves mood and alertness, reduces stress, enhances cognitive function, boosts energy levels.

41. Oil Diffusers

- *Description:* Use oil diffusers to disperse essential oils into the air.
- *Benefits:* Promotes relaxation, reduces stress and anxiety, improves mood, enhances respiratory health.

42. Personal Trainer

- *Description:* Work with a personal trainer to create a fitness plan.
- *Benefits:* Improves fitness level, boosts motivation, provides personalized guidance, enhances physical health.

43. DIY Beauty Treatments

- *Description:* Make your own natural beauty treatments.

- *Benefits:* Improves skin health, promotes relaxation, enhances self-care routine, boosts self-confidence.

44. Read Bible

- *Description:* Read the Bible for spiritual nourishment.

- *Benefits:* Enhances spiritual well-being, provides guidance and wisdom, promotes peace of mind, reduces stress.

45. Playing an Instrument

- *Description:* Play a musical instrument.

- *Benefits:* Reduces stress, enhances cognitive function, improves hand-eye coordination, boosts mood.

46. Riding Horses

    - *Description:* Engage in horseback riding.

    - *Benefits:* Reduces stress, improves balance and coordination, promotes relaxation, enhances mood.

47. Sleeping In

    - *Description:* Allow yourself to sleep in occasionally.

    - *Benefits:* Improves mood, reduces stress, enhances cognitive function, promotes overall well-being.

48. Minding My Own Business

    - *Description:* Focus on your own life and avoid unnecessary drama.

    - *Benefits:* Reduces stress, promotes inner peace, enhances focus and productivity, improves relationships.

49. Take Yourself on a Date

- *Description:* Treat yourself to a solo outing.

- *Benefits:* Promotes self-love and self-care, boosts mood, enhances independence, provides a sense of empowerment.

50. Travel

- *Description:* Travel to new destinations or revisit favorite places.

- *Benefits:* Promotes relaxation, reduces stress, enhances creativity, provides new experiences and perspectives.

51. Wash and Condition Hair

- *Description:* Wash and condition your hair using products suited to

- *Benefits:* Improves hair health, enhances appearance, promotes relaxation, boosts self-confidence.

CHAPTER 14

CONCLUSION

EMBRACING YOUR JOURNEY OF SELF-NURTURING FINAL THOUGHTS

As we come to the end of this journey together, I want to congratulate you on taking the time to nurture yourself. The path to self-care and self-nurturing is not always easy, but it is incredibly rewarding. By prioritizing your well-being and making self-care a priority, you have taken an important step towards living a more fulfilling and balanced life.

Throughout this book, we have explored various aspects of self-nurturing, from understanding the importance of self-care to practical tips for nurturing your body, mind, and spirit. We have discussed the challenges you may face, such as finding time for self-care and overcoming obstacles, and we have provided strategies to help you navigate these challenges.

Encouragement to Keep Nurturing Yourself

As you continue on your journey of self-nurturing, I encourage you to be gentle with yourself. Self-care is not about perfection; it's about progress. There will be days when you may struggle to prioritize your well-being, and that's okay. Remember that self-care is a lifelong journey, and it's important to be patient and kind to yourself along the way.

I also encourage you to stay connected to your why. Why is self-nurturing important to you? What are the benefits you hope to gain from prioritizing your well-being? By staying connected to your why, you can stay motivated and focused on your goals, even when faced with challenges.

Acknowledgments

I would like to take a moment to acknowledge and thank all those who have supported me in my creative part of my journey in this thing called life. To my family who have always supported every dream, goal and desire I have ever had ~ I love you! To my real friends who allow me a safe space to just be ~ I value you! Thank you all for your love, encouragement, and understanding. To my editor and best friend since the 3rd grade, Kimberly Cousins, Owner of Write Touch Publications, thank you for constantly encouraging me to write.

Thank you to each client that has trusted me with your bodies inside of your fitness journey. I don't take that lightly. Your strength and passion to become the best inspires me to be the best trainer, coach, and motivator I can be.

And finally, to you, the reader, thank you for joining me on this journey. I hope that this book has inspired you to prioritize your well-being and to Normalize Nurturing U in a way that honors who you are and who you were destined to be.

In conclusion, I want to leave you with this final thought:

You are deserving of love, care, and nurture. By prioritizing your well-being and making self-care a priority, you are taking an important step towards living

In conclusion, I want to a more fulfilling and balanced life. leave you with this final

Embrace your journey of self-nurturing, thought: and remember that you are worthy of all the love and care in the world. You are deserving of love, care, and nurture. By prioritizing your well-being and making self-care a priority, you are taking an important step towards living a more fulfilling and balanced life. Embrace your journey of self-nurturing, and remember that you are worthy of all the love and care in the world.

PAULA MARIE

Paula Marie

BlackGirlsDoPilates2

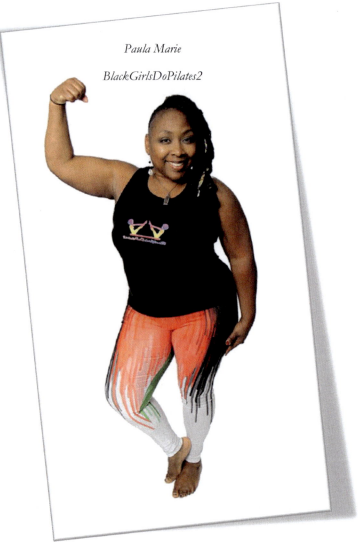

Made in the USA
Middletown, DE
28 May 2024

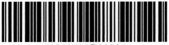